TESTOSTERONE

How To Boost Your Testosterone Naturally

ROBIN DABAS

CONTENTS

ACKNOWLEDGMENTS

I would like to thank all of you men and women out there who are taking your health in your own hands, by reading this book not only will you boost your testosterone naturally, but you will learn and apply new things that will change your life for the better. I wish you all good health on your journey's and hope what's in this book help's and benefits you, as much as it has for myself and others around me.

Thank you to the cover designer for taking my vision and creating it for me in this wonderful cover you see now.

I would also like to give a special thanks to my mother and father who have given me the strength and courage to push myself out of my comfort zone, so that I can reach greater heights and achieve the dreams that I truly desire. They stuck by me and supported me when times were tough, their love, and support has truly made me the man I am today. I will always love and cherish you in my heart.

I would also like to dedicate this book to my baby Prince, my fury four-legged friend. Who was the most loving and loyal creature anyone could ask for. May you rest in peace.

INTRODUCTION

Testosterone, the one and only male hormone that make's us men of any age feel and look better? Are you sick and tired of being sick and tired, not getting the results in the gym? Are you unable to get or maintain an erection? Have your testicle's shrunk? Are you experiencing hair loss? Not feeling yourself? These may be signs that you have low T.

There are natural scientifically researched ways of boosting your testosterone to their optimal levels. By taking the necessary steps outlined in this book you will be well on your way to boosting your testosterone. You don't need to be on testosterone replacement therapy or any other form of unnatural intervention. What is proposed in this book is research backed natural ways of increasing your testosterone levels.

This book was written with the intention of giving you a life worth living. Giving you the health, vitality, energy, and outlook on life that you were meant to have. Take back control and master your T.

WHAT IS TESTOSTERONE? AND WHY WE AS MEN NEED THIS HORMONE IN HIGHER QUANTITIES

Testosterone has often been referred to as the most important hormone in males. In fact, that's exactly how the National Institutes of Health describes it.

While it is a hormone that is found in both males and females, testosterone is found in higher quantities in males, and plays a vital role in sexual and reproductive development. It also helps in other areas such as bone and muscle mass and red blood cell production.

Testosterone is a powerful hormone that begins to increase in production during puberty for males, and then taper off after men turn 30 years old. It's no wonder, then, that the peak in male sexual virility and performance is usually associated with teens and men in their 20s. It's because of the higher production of testosterone that this happens.

Testosterone is such a powerful hormone that lower levels of it can affect people in more ways than just lower sexual desire and performance. In fact, low levels of testosterone can be associated with thinner bones, weight gain, lower energy and feelings of depression. That's why it's essential that testosterone levels are kept in check and stable throughout a male's life.

Before one can understand how to check for testosterone levels, the dangers of low levels and what may cause it, one needs to first understand exactly what testosterone is and how it works in the body.

What is testosterone and what are hormones, exactly?

Testosterone is a hormone that is characterized in the class of androgens, which also includes steroids and anabolic steroids. As such, testosterone is extremely powerful. Just think of what steroids do to body builders and other athletes, or even the power they possess when they're prescribed for health conditions such as asthma, pneumonia and other illnesses.

There are two types of testosterone that are found in the bloodstream. Bound testosterone accounts for almost all the testosterone in your body, around 98 percent of it to be exact. Bound testosterone means it's literally bound to other things in your body, but mainly either the protein albumin or the protein sex hormone binding globulin.

The other 2 percent of testosterone found in your body is called free testosterone, or free T. This type of testosterone works exactly the opposite way of bound testosterone – it is not chemically bound to anything else in your body. It roams freely about.

Different hormones are produced in the body for a number of functions, both in males and females. According to the Hormone Health Network, these chemicals are messengers created in the endocrine glands, and hormones "control most major bodily functions, from simple basic needs like hunger to complex systems like reproduction, and even the emotions and mood."

Each class of hormone is produced in a different gland in the body, and is responsible for a different task. Some of the main glands are the pancreas, which produces insulin that helps control blood sugar; the thyroid, which produces hormones that help with heart rate and burning calories; the hypothalamus, which regulates body temperature, hunger and moods; and the pituitary, known as the "master control gland," that takes control of other glands and produces growth-triggering hormones.

While each hormone plays a vital role in keeping the balance of a healthy body, there are a few that stand out above the rest. Cortisol, which is produced in the adrenal gland, assists the body in the ways it responds to stress, which is why it's often referred to as the "stress hormone." This is an essential role that helps keep the body in check during stressful situations, which helps keep blood pressure and heart rate low when the surroundings around us aren't always peachy.

Testosterone is a major hormone in both men and women, but especially so for men. It's produced in the testes for men, while women's testosterone is produced in the ovaries.

Hormones in general are responsible for key functions inside our body. When our glands are producing these hormones at just the right levels, our body is able to perform at peak levels in a healthy way. It's sort of like an orchestra.

Think of each gland as a separate section in the orchestra. The testes could be the brass section, for example. The adrenal gland could be the woodwinds. The pituitary could be percussion, and so on. Then, each hormone in the gland "section" could represent a different musical position. Testosterone could be the lead trumpet and cortisol could be lead clarinet, and so on and so forth.

When each section (or gland, in this example) of the orchestra is performing at top-notch level, that means that each musical position (or hormone) is performing at his or her best. And when each person in each section of the orchestra is performing his or her best all at the same time, the end result is a beautiful musical masterpiece for the orchestra (or the human body, in our terms).

Hormones are so powerful and so important that, much like a single player in the orchestra, if one thing is off or if one hormone or gland isn't performing properly, it can have serious effects for the rest of the body, and not just in the ways you might think.

What does testosterone do?

As we've discussed already, testosterone is the main sex hormone in men. Its primary responsibility is to produce sperm in the testicles. Healthy sperm, as we all know, is an essential component in the reproductive process. Without healthy sperm, it is impossible to reproduce.

Testosterone production begins in the pituitary gland near the base of the brain, and while it is being produced, it creates signals of sexual desire in men. While men produce some level of testosterone in just about every stage of their life, the tipping point stage of this production – and when it is at its highest level – occurs at the start of puberty.

Puberty is the stage in life when a boy begins to grow into a man, both figuratively and literally. From an anatomical stand-point, a boy's body begins to undergo some dramatic changes, and most of these changes are due to the increased production of testosterone in the body. Any boy knows that when he begins to hit puberty, typically in the early teenage years, things start happening to the body that haven't happened up until this point, at least not as dramatically as they are now.

The increased production of testosterone in a boy's body at the start of puberty contributes to what is often the beginning of his first true growth spurt. It's why you see a lot of boys in their early teenage years begin to grow in height, sometimes quite substantially in a short amount of time, depending on their genetic make-up. In addition, a boy's body will begin to see increased strength in bones and muscles. This is a major reason why, even without increased exercise or weight training, boys might start "filling out" their frame, as it's often referred to, and lose what is often called that "baby fat."

The other effects of the increased production of testosterone at this stage in a boy's life are the ones that are more well-known. These include a deepening of the voice, the growth of facial, pubic and body hair, and the growth of both the penis and the testicles.

During puberty, the body begins to produce testosterone at these higher levels because it is a time when the body needs to start transitioning, from a hormonal perspective, from a boy to a man. This is not to say that increased testosterone production at puberty makes a boy into a man from a figurative perspective. Any mother and father of a boy going through puberty will certainly attest to that fact. However, from just a medical point of view, puberty is the official starting point to the body's transition from a boy to a man, bringing with it adult-like appearance, sound and function.

While testosterone production begins to increase dramatically during puberty, it produces at high levels for most males through the age of 30, at which time it begins to taper off somewhat (we'll hit on this in more depth later). After puberty, testosterone still plays a vital role in the health of a man's body. While it continues to contribute to sex drive and sperm production, essential functions through the time in a man's life when he's most likely to begin producing offspring, it also plays a huge role in continued facial and body hair growth, muscle mass and strength, bone density, fat distribution and the production of red blood cells.

That's why continued, healthy production of testosterone is essential for a male's body even after the production of it begins to reduce after the age of 30. Some men might think that it's not as important to have healthy levels of testosterone once they are either finished having children or make the decision to not have children any more. Older men might especially think it's not as important, as producing offspring might be the last thing on their mind, and they might be tired of shaving multiple times a week anyway. There also isn't as much of a negative stigma associated with male pattern baldness as it is with women losing the hair on their head.

But as we'll soon learn, having lower (or even higher) levels of testosterone at any stage in life is not a good thing, and can have dramatic ill effects if not recognized and treated properly.

Why do men need more testosterone?

While testosterone is present in women and is a necessary hormone for their development, men need much more testosterone to lead a healthy life. In fact, as Very Well Health says, "healthy males who have gone through puberty have 20 times the levels of testosterone compared to a healthy female."

Too much testosterone for women can cause infertility. In men, it works both ways, as too little or too much testosterone can result in having low sperm counts, which could then cause fertility issues with men.

While testosterone acts in some different ways for both males and females, it also acts in other ways the same for both genders. Normal testosterone levels are essential because the hormone may help regulate pain tolerance, and aids in learning, memory and cognitive empathy, research has found.

Testosterone is specifically associated with spatial intelligence, and men with abnormally low levels of the hormone are often at risk for learning disabilities. In another sense, too much testosterone may contribute to one having trouble reading the emotions of another person. Researchers believe this is one reason why women as a whole are considered more empathetic and better at this skill, because they have much lower levels of testosterone than men. Think about that one next time you come across an instance of "women's intuition."

Total testosterone and free testosterone levels can be up to 30 times greater in healthy males over the age of 19 compared to healthy females of the same age. An interesting aspect of testosterone between the genders is that infant boys and girls have the same amount of testosterone. It isn't until boys hit puberty that they begin to produce more testosterone than girls at the same stage.

This happens because males need more testosterone to produce sperm than women do for reproductive functions, plus the extra testosterone also helps contribute to building more muscle mass. And in an anatomically-historical aspect, men need more toned muscles – need to be stronger, to say it another way - than women. In the old days – like the really, really old days of hunters and gatherers – men did the literal heavy lifting, so they needed more muscle mass to handle the greater weight-bearing tasks.

The levels of testosterone that males need also helps contribute to their sex drive, which, again, from a simply physical standpoint, is needed in the ingrained human need to reproduce.

It's never good to have too much or too little of anything, and that is especially true for testosterone in men. Most men who suffer from an unbalanced testosterone level check in on the low end of testosterone. That's because testosterone levels peak at around age 20 for men. In addition, researchers have found that men could experience a 1 percent drop in their testosterone levels each year between ages 30 and 50.

Sometimes, this annual drop doesn't even show up on a male body's radar. Other times, the gradual drop could cause complications in men, especially around age 60 or afterward. In fact, this decrease in testosterone could cause a condition called hypogonadism, often referred to as andropause or "male menopause."

Low-T levels could be the result of other causes as well, not just the normal annual drop in the body's natural production rate. Low testosterone could be the result of a testicular injury; of taking too many opiate medications; of hormonal disorders; of chronic diseases such as type 2 diabetes, kidney and liver diseases, and obesity; and of genetic diseases such as myotonic dystrophy, Klinefelter syndrome and Kallman syndrome.

No matter what the causes are, the effects of having low-T levels, especially for males, can be serious. Low testosterone levels could result in a decline in energy, strength, stamina and mental aggressiveness. These are not good things when talking about performance in the bedroom, but also outside of it, as well.

In addition to a decline in sex drive and trouble getting erec-

11

tions, plenty of men with low-T levels experience more aches and pains in bones and joints, a gain of weight and possibly even osteoporosis – a fragile bone condition that could cause bones to break rather easily.

So while most of testosterone's rep is as the male hormone that contributes to sex and sexual desire, not having enough of it could be dangerous for men in other ways. TV commercials and other advertisements for low-T levels focus mostly on the sexual aspects of the condition – just think of those "little blue pill" commercials that focus on older men and what would seem to be their desire to have relations with their partners. That's all fine and dandy, because it is a true result of low T levels.

However, it may also be a reason why a lot of males don't get their testosterone levels checked out or, when they do, why they don't seek further treatment. Studies have shown that as recently as 2011, an estimated 13 million men in the United States had low-T issues. Since 2012, the number of older men diagnosed with low-T levels increased 170 percent. The problem, though, is that only about 5 percent to 10 percent of men who have low-T seek treatment for it.

Possibly because of the sexual stigma associated with low testosterone levels that is promulgated by these marketing campaigns, and the common misperception that low-T levels mean someone isn't a "full man," men often don't take their levels of testosterone seriously, or they're ashamed when they are found to have low-T levels. But males shouldn't feel ashamed if they have low-T levels. It's common enough in today's world, plus it's a hormone imbalance that could cause plenty of complications and health risks, as we've already discussed.

Medically, low-T levels as a result of aging is now officially recognized as late-onset hypogonadism. This ailment is associated with, obviously, sexual dysfunction as well as metabolic and cardiovascular diseases. It can also cause mood changes, reduced cognitive function, fatigue, depressions, anger, skin changes and a decrease in bone mass and bone mineral density. It's not something that anyone would want, but it's something that more and more older men are experiencing, especially with life expectancy rates continuing to increase.

The good news is that testosterone levels can be tested through simple bloodwork that measures the amount of hormone in the blood. If low-T levels are found, patients can easily be prescribed testosterone "therapy" in various forms of medication. These forms can be a gel that gets applied to the upper arms, shoulders or abdomen each day, or a skin patch put on the body twice a day; or injections every two to three weeks, or implants that last four two six months.

Testosterone therapy has proven to raise low-T levels in the body, researchers have found, which helps contribute to greater strength, cognitive functions and even sex drive as well.

The point of all of this is that having healthy, normal, regulated testosterone levels is essential for the male body to function, and not just from a sexual perspective. That's why it is very important for men to get their testosterone levels tested by a doctor regularly, especially as they continue to age after 30, or if they are having issues with their sex drive at a younger age. Testing for T levels can be done through a simple blood sample, so no need to fret about anything complicated, expensive or intrusive.

Like any other disease, ailment or condition, the sooner and more often you identify an imbalance in your testosterone level, the easier it will be to correct the imbalance, and the less damage it will have also possibly caused to your body to that point. So don't worry about the stigma associated with testosterone levels and sexual performance.

The importance of having healthy testosterone levels at all ages for all males is more important than the potential embarrassment of testing for an imbalance and getting treated to get your hormone levels back to their proper place.

THE TESTOSTERONE BOOSTING BENEFITS OF BORON & ITS SYMBIOTIC RELATIONSHIP WITH VITAMIN D

M any men are faced with the challenge of low testosterone levels, especially as they get older. Low-T levels are a concern for many men, not just because testosterone contributes to essential reproductive functions and sex drive, but also because healthy testosterone levels help prevent against the thinning of bones, weight gain, lower energy and feelings of depressions.

There are many reasons why men could be experiencing low-T levels, but perhaps the most common reason is a natural one: Starting around age 30, testosterone levels in men decrease by about 1 percent each year. This natural decreasing in testosterone doesn't always manifest itself as an issue for men, but when it does, there are serious potential consequences if it's not addressed properly.

With the negative stigma around low-T levels subsiding in today's culture, testosterone-boosting products are flooding the market, promising a proven cure for low-T levels and a healthy regulation of the essential hormone. With all these fancy products and choices out there, perhaps two of the more effective supplements in doing so are interconnected ones that occur naturally in our food and the environment around us – boron and vitamin D.

We all know what vitamin D is. Vitamin D is an essential vitamin that's found in many of our foods, such as fortified milk, fatty fish and egg yolks, and also in sunlight. But many of us aren't as up-to-date on where boron is found, or, more likely, many of us have never even heard of boron before. So what is it? Where is it found? What are its benefits? And how do you get it?

What is boron and what are its benefits?

Boron is a trace mineral and micronutrient that plays many vital roles in both humans and in nature. It is especially important in the process of metabolism for not just humans but also plants and animals.

Boron works by increasing magnesium and vitamin D serum levels in the blood. Both magnesium and vitamin D are known to have a positive effect on testosterone levels by either producing the raw material needed for the production of testosterone, or by supporting the other structures involved in the production of testosterone. So by increasing both magnesium and vitamin D levels, boron is effectively boosting testosterone quite substantially.

Most of us are getting some level of boron in our diets every day, even if we aren't making a conscious effort to do so. Some of the foods with the highest level of boron are nuts such as almond, hazelnuts, walnuts and Brazil nuts, and other foods such as raisins, dried apricots, red kidney beans and dates.

According to a study published in the U.S. National Library of Medicine, boron has been proven as an important trace mineral, in part "because it (1) is essential for the growth and maintenance of bone; (2) greatly improves wound healing; (3) beneficially impacts the body's use of estrogen, testosterone, and vitamin D; (4) boost magnesium absorption," among many other reasons. The study focused primarily on "boron's most salient effects on human health, including its impact on bone development and regeneration, wound healing, the production of metabolism and sex steroids and vitamin D, and the absorption and use of calcium and magnesium."

Boron's important role in metabolism and other functions in the body is due to the way it handles calcium, magnesium and phosphorus. In addition to these benefits, boric acid, which is made from boron, has been used by women to kill yeast that can cause vaginal infections. Boron itself is also thought to have antioxidant properties, helping to kill "free radicals" and other toxins in the body.

One of boron's most important roles is in protecting joints and bones. Boron induces the mineralization activity known as osteoblasts, a type of cell that creates new material to build bones. That's why it's also closely linked to speeding up wound healing, in a way, with a 1990 study revealing that boric acid treatment on deep wounds could reduce the overall healing time by two-thirds. That's quite powerful stuff.

Boron also helps to keep your teeth and gums healthy since it helps reduce inflammation throughout the body. And, surprisingly, good oral health is essential to have healthy sex hormones. Furthermore, boron helps block excess estrogen, increases muscle and bone strength, improves mental clarity and muscle coordination, reduces inflammation and helps treat arthritis.

But boron is getting the most publicity today because of its role in helping to regulate and maintain levels of hormones, especially estrogen and testosterone. The mineral is important for both men and women, and it has been proven to boost both of these hormones, in both men and women. Increased levels of testosterone in men can be a good thing, especially if one has low-T levels, but increased production of estrogen usually is not, which is why it's essential that people who take boron as a supplement are careful with how it's affecting their body in particular. If your intake of boron is increasing your levels of estrogen too much, then it will be necessary to adjust the amount of intake to regulate the levels of estrogen versus testosterone.

Boron and testosterone levels are so interlinked that a boron deficiency could also lead to a sex hormone imbalance. So a lack of boron could lead to a lack of testosterone and an increase in the negative effects that such a situation could cause.

The testosterone-boosting effects of boron

While boron as a testosterone-boosting supplement hasn't been researched as much as other vitamins and minerals, it has been proven to increase T levels when taken as a daily supplement. One study in particular found that taking boron increased testosterone levels by 28.3 percent within seven days. That's quite a significant increase and one that could do wonders for those suffering from low testosterone.

This large increase was found in free testosterone levels in the body, but it also found that after taking a 10 mg daily supplement of boron for four weeks, overall testosterone levels increased by 11.4 percent as well. Free testosterone makes up only about 2 percent of a person's overall testosterone levels. The rest is called bound testosterone, which means the hormone is literally bound to a different element in the body. Free testosterone, therefore, is not bound to anything else.

In addition, boron helps counteract what is sometimes an ill-fated side effect of increasing testosterone levels. When testosterone levels go up, so, too, do levels of sex hormone binding globulin, also known as SHBG. The bad part about SHBG is that it binds to sex hormones and can therefore prevent their effects. That's not a good thing, obviously, especially in men who have low-T levels and need all the powers that more testosterone can give them.

Boron increases testosterone levels by increasing the concentration of steroid hormones in the blood. Testosterone, remember, is part of a hormone class called androgens, which also includes steroids and anabolic steroids. So the more steroid hormones that are in the blood, the more testosterone that will be present as well.

However, in addition to actually increasing levels of testosterone, taking boron as a supplement can also reduce SHBG levels in the blood, which in turn can allow the extra testosterone in your body to actually do the job you're it's supposed to do. Some have suggested that this could be a reason why boron was found to have a greater increase in free testosterone than on overall testosterone in the body – because it will not bind to anything else.

Another recent study actually found that people who have low testosterone levels and also low levels of boron in their diet could benefit more from taking a boron supplement than people who do not have low-T and boron levels. In these cases, testosterone levels were shown to increase more than two-fold with a daily regimen of a boron supplement.

Increased testosterone levels are proven to help build strong bones and joints, and boron itself has similar effects. That's why ensuring your diet is sufficient in boron, or adding a supplement to your daily intake, could work doubly good in this area.

One study looked at patients with confirmed osteoporotic disease, and found that half the patients reported improvements with their symptoms by taking a dose of only 6 mg of boron a day. The boron can do this directly all by itself, but the fact that it also increases testosterone levels – which also has bone and joint improvement properties – makes it even more effective.

Yet another comprehensive study looked at the comparative effects of daily and weekly boron supplements. The study wanted to examine the effects of acute boron intake on males. The participants of the study were given a 10-milligram supplement of boron every day for a week, and regular blood tests to monitor the effects.

The results found that the supplements caused a "significant increase" in testosterone levels. It also found that the supplements "caused an increase in Dihydrotestosterone (DHT), a hormone responsible for manly traits and vitamin D, which is required for producing testosterone."

Other impressive effects of the supplement intake observed were a drop in female hormone estradiol and, as mentioned before, the sex hormone binding globulin (SHBG). Finally, the study found that the 10-milligram dosage of boron supplement daily caused an increase in levels of cortisol, which is the stress hormone responsible for keeping us calm, cool and collected in pressure-packed situations.

What does vitamin D have to do with testosterone and boron?

Vitamin D is well-known to have a positive effect on fertility, and this now goes not just for reproductive health in a woman's body, but also in relation to a man's sexual health. And that's because vitamin D seems to have a positive effect on increasing testosterone levels.

A study showed that people who took 50nmol/L of serum vitamin D daily for one year reported an average 25.2 percent increase in testosterone levels. Like boron, vitamin D isn't naturally found in too many foods, limited mainly to seafood, milk and some juices. However, you can also get vitamin D by simply catching some rays from the sun. The problem is that many people have lower-than-needed levels of vitamin D in their body, even if they are exposed to enough sun.

Vitamin D by itself has many health benefits. Vitamin D helps absorb calcium and promotes bone growth. If you don't have enough vitamin D, you may experience a softness in your bones. A vitamin D deficiency has also been linked to breast, colon and prostate cancers, heart disease, depression and weight gain.

Having healthy levels of vitamin D is essential for a healthy, productive body. And maintaining that healthy level of vitamin D is very important for long-term, sufficient testosterone levels.

A recent German study found that vitamin D does have a testosterone-boosting effect. The great part about this study, for those who have low-T levels at least, is that it was not conducted to find out whether vitamin D had this power or not; it was just a separate finding that occurred. The study, in fact, was studying weight loss and not levels of testosterone. So the fact that the testosterone levels increased is a great result for low-T patients, as the researchers weren't controlling the environment to try to prove, or disprove, vitamin D's effects on testosterone levels.

What the study found in relation to testosterone is that testicles have receptors for vitamin D, which the researches said suggests that vitamin D plays a role in healthy testosterone production. They also found a definitive link between levels of vitamin D and levels of testosterone in the blood. The researchers also referred to a previous study on mice, which found that mice who did not have receptors for vitamin D had much lower levels of testosterone than those that did.

The amazing thing about boron is that, in addition to boosting levels of testosterone in your system, it also helps prevent vitamin D deficiency. It does this by increasing the half-life and bioavailability of vitamin D. This means that boron helps to increase the amount of time that vitamin D stays in a useful state in your body before the body naturally filters it out with other waste.

As the U.S. National Library of Medicine states: "Boron's beneficial effects on bone metabolism are due in part to the roles it plays in both producing E2 and in increasing its biological half-life and that of vitamin D." E2, for clarification, is estradiol, an estrogen steroid hormone, which is the major female sex hormone.

A study conducted by the University of Wisconsin-Madison showed that when boron was given to rats with a vitamin D deficiency, bone ash increased 5.8 percent over only an eight-week period. This is significant, as it means their bones were much stronger as a result of the increased amount of bone mass.

Yet another study of clinically diagnosed patients with low vitamin D levels were given 6 milligrams of boron for 60 days. The results? That not only did the participants' DHEA levels increase by an average of 56 percent, but their free testosterone levels increased by an average of 29.5 percent as well!

This goes back to what we talked about before in how boron boosts testosterone levels. Most of the times, when you take products to boost your testosterone levels, you end up increasing the amount of sex hormone binding globulin (SHBG) as well. This increases your overall testosterone levels, but not your free testosterone, since the SHBG binds to it. Since boron effectively blocks SHBG in the blood, the end result is a boost in free testosterone levels, and not overall testosterone levels.

Boron and vitamin D work hand-in-hand to support a lot of essential functions in the body and prevent many diseases and ailments. The mineral and vitamin work hand-in-hand like a perfect dynamic duo. It's as if boron is acting like Batman who leads the way but needs his trusty sidekick Robin (or vitamin D in this scenario) to save the day and keep Gotham (or your body) safe.

It's a big domino effect that starts by making sure your body is getting enough boron on a daily basis. First, boron acts as a protectant, extending the effectiveness of vitamin D in your body. Then, boron goes to work as an actor itself, ensuring the body is properly absorbing other essential minerals. When all the dominos have fallen, the end result is an increased level of testosterone.

This is especially important because, like boron, vitamin D isn't found in very many food naturally. It's a fat-soluble nutrient that is contained in mushrooms and fatty fish naturally, and that is added to milk. The body can also get extra vitamin D with exposure to the sun, but the challenge is that too much exposure to the sun can be very harmful to the skin if it's not protected.

That's why many people who have a vitamin D deficiency are forced to take a supplement to regulate their levels. And it's yet another reason why boron is so important to testosterone levels, allowing the vitamin D that you do have in your body to last longer and be more effective.

So how do you get more boron?

Now that we know how good boron is for your body, and how much it can help stabilize your levels of vitamin D and increase your levels of testosterone, the question becomes, how can you get more of it? The thing is that your body doesn't produce any boron on its own, so the only way to get it is to consume it.

Dried fruits and nuts are some of the best sources of boron. In addition to the food sources we mentioned earlier, you can also get good levels of boron by consuming Shiraz Cabernet wine, lentils, chickpeas, peaches, celery, red grapes, honey, olives, red apples, pears, broccoli and carrots.

The issue, though, is that even in the foods in which boron is most prevalently found, there isn't a heck of a lot of boron in it. Avocados are a great example of this. An entire cup of avocados only contacts about 1.7 milligrams of boron. If you're eating avocados as a way to boost your testosterone levels, you would need to eat approximately five avocados every day to get the desired result.

Like any other mineral, you can also get boron by taking a daily supplement. Doctors recommend that if you take a boron supplement, you take something with at least 3 millgrams but up to as many as 10 milligrams. This can be done in one of two ways. You can either take a daily multi-vitamin that has that amount of boron in it, or you can take a boron pill such as boric acid as part of your daily routine.

While there is no official recommended daily dosage of boron, according to the U.S. National Institutes of Health, the organization does say that adult males shouldn't take more than 20 mg of boron per day by mouth. After all, too much of anything is never good a thing.

That being said, there are no long-term proven side effects of taking a boron supplement, and boron toxicity rarely happens because the body is able to dispel the mineral rather quickly.

Males who have low testosterone levels are constantly searching for effective ways at increasing their T levels. And while there are different gels, patches, injections and other treatments on the market that could help to increase testosterone levels, there are also proven natural ways that you can do so as well.

Including a daily regimen of boron into your diet through boron-rich foods or through a boron supplement is a highly suggested way to increase your testosterone levels. Boron, combined with healthy vitamin D intake, could get you well on your way to having a healthier, stable level of testosterone in your body.

HOW ZINC CAN BOOST YOUR IMMUNITY AS WELL AS YOUR TESTOSTERONE

No one likes getting sick. It can be an uncomfortable feeling, at the very least, with alternating feelings of hot and cold, sweaty and dry, thirst, upset stomach, headaches and watery eyes. It can be severe, too, with extreme nausea, body aches and pains, and high temperatures that are dangerous for the body.

We all want to avoid getting sick, and the best way to do so is to live the healthiest life we can live. That means eating right, exercising, clearing our minds of stress and getting a restful night's sleep every night. But even the healthiest people in the world get sick at times. There are plenty of harmful germs and bacteria that live in our world all around us, and sometimes these germs and bacteria enter our body and aren't warded off fast enough to prevent us from getting sick.

The immune system is our body's line of defense against viruses, bacteria, parasites and other harmful things that could enter the body and cause things to get out of whack. The immune system works throughout the entire body, as it is a system made up of cells, organs, proteins and tissues that work hand-in-hand to protect our body by recognizing what is supposed to be in there and what is not. When a foreign substance – like a virus or bacteria – is found, the immune system gets to work to expel the foreign object.

The immune system kicks into high gear at times like these, doing its best to attack the foreign substance and get the body regulated again before too much damage is done. A high body temperature, runny nose, cough and other symptoms of a common cold, for example, are all either ways the immune system changes your body to dispel the harmful material, or side effects of doing so.

Without a healthy and properly working immune system, your body wouldn't have the ability to fight off even the common cold, which could lead to more serious ailments such as pneumonia. That's why it's important, for example, to be careful with germs and environments for people with compromised immune systems such as the elderly or not-fully-developed immune systems such as infants.

Like all other aspects of the body, the immune system runs at full capacity for most people as long as they are taking care of the body as a whole, paying attention to what they put into it in terms of food, beverages and other toxins, and how they treat it in the form of exercise, stress management and sleep.

But there are also proven ways to help boost the function of your immune system through natural supplements of vitamins and minerals. One of the most well-known immune-boosting supplement is vitamin C, which is found naturally in citrus fruits, among other things. Go to your local pharmacy or drug store and you're certain to find cold and flu remedies and immune system boosting supplements touting the power of vitamin C. Those products are not misleading; vitamin C is, indeed, a powerful supplement for boosting immune system function.

A lesser-known, yet equally as powerful, immune system booster, and one that could have healthy benefits in other areas of your body, is zinc. In fact, zinc is essential to a healthy immune system, and a deficiency of zinc can make a person much more susceptible to disease and illness.

Zinc has yet another powerful effect, as well. It has been proven to not only boost testosterone, but regulate its levels as well. Studies have linked a zinc deficiency to lower testosterone levels. So making sure you have enough zinc in your diet, and supplementing it with zinc in other forms if you do not, can have powerful effects on not only your immune system but your testosterone levels as well.

What is zinc?

Zinc is a trace element in the body that is responsible for a number of different important functions, helping to stimulate the activity of at least 100 different enzymes. Zinc is extremely powerful, too, as your body doesn't need a lot of it to perform at tip-top shape. In fact, doctors recommend that women only need 8 milligrams a day in their diet, while men are recommended to have 11 milligrams a day.

Zinc is an important part of having a nutritious diet. A zinc deficiency can lead to growth impediments in children, lower levels of testosterone in men and a higher susceptibility to disease and illness in everyone. Zinc's role for a healthy immune system is "correctly synthesizing DNA, promoting healthy growth during childhood and healing wounds," according to Medical News Today.

Zinc helps control and regulate immune responses and even

attacks infected or cancerous cells. As a result, a zinc deficiency can "severely impair immune system function."

Various studies have also found that zinc can have a powerful effect on preventing acne, treating attention deficit hyperactivity disorder (ADHD), osteoporosis, and preventing and treating pneumonia. Zinc helps with reducing the risk of inflammatory diseases, can help prevent age-related macular degeneration, can boost learning and memory, can treat diarrhea, and plays a significant role in wound healing.

It's obvious that zinc has vast benefits on our entire bodies, but for the purposes of staying focused, we'll concentrate on two major areas: the immune system and testosterone.

How zinc boosts immune system function

Studies have shown that adequate levels of zinc in the body are essential for a properly-functioning immune system, and zinc supplements can even help boost the immune system in extra times of need, such as when one is experiencing a sickness or disease. But how does zinc actually work in this regard?

Researchers from Ohio State University have found that a protein in the body "lures zinc into key cells that are first-responders against infection. The zinc then interacts with a process that is vital to the fight against infection and by doing so helps balance the immune response."

This research showed that zinc's role in fighting disease and sickness is a very active one. It's not a passive player in the fight, just sitting back and providing support to other elements of the immune system. Rather, it is an active participant that goes to work directly to fight against the bad stuff in our body.

The study found that zinc's role in fighting disease and sickness isn't to actually cure the disease or sickness, but rather to cut it off at the path and stop it in its tracks. This then allows the other aspects of the immune system to go hard at work to rid the body of the harmful elements, without having to worry that things could get out of hand and force the body to enter panic mode. Zinc, then, is a damage controller in the process of fighting off disease and sickness.

The researcher's of this study also believe that a lack of zinc when the body needs it in times of disease and sickness, at the onset of the infection, can lead to serious consequences such as excessive inflammation. Some inflammation at these times is good, as it helps to ward off the disease or sickness, but too much of it can lead to more serious consequences in the body. That's why scientists believe that taking zinc tablets at the onset of the infection has proven to be effective at stopping the attack on the body in its tracks.

Daren Knoell, a senior author of the study and a professor of pharmacy and internal medicine at Ohio State University, said this about zinc's power, according to an article in Science Daily:

"Without zinc on board to begin with, it could increase vulnerability to infection. But our work is focused on what happens once you get an infection – if you are deficient in zinc you are at a disadvantage because your defense system is amplified, and inappropriately so. The benefit to health is explicit: Zinc is beneficial because it stops the action of a protein, ultimately preventing excess inflammation."

The benefit is "explicit," he said. That's a rather poignant and powerful statement.

To sum up everything in more common terms, the presence of healthy levels of zinc in the body before an infection occurs is important to keeping an overall healthy immune system, functioning properly on a daily basis. And when an infection does occur, increasing your intake of zinc will help to stop an infection in its path, to make sure that the disease, virus or sickness does not progress any worse than it already has.

What is zinc's relation to testosterone?

Zinc levels and testosterone levels are very much intertwined. For years, scientists have known that adequate zinc levels have been associated with reproductive health. A zinc deficiency has been linked to lower sperm quality in men, for example, as one study found that subjects had a higher sperm count after taking a supplement of zinc sulfate and folic acid. Similarly, another study found that a zinc deficiency could be a risk factor for low quality of sperm and male infertility.

Low levels of zinc in your body can lead to low levels of testosterone in your body. As such, maintaining an adequate level of zinc in your body, and/or taking a zinc supplement if needed, can help raise your testosterone levels.

Research suggests that zinc affects testosterone levels because it may affect the cells in the testes that produce testosterone. Remember that zinc plays an important role in helping enzymes break down food and other nutrients as well as building proteins and promoting cell health.

A recent study found that men who received 30 milligrams of zinc per day had increased levels of free testosterone in their bodies. A zinc supplement can be especially effective for men with low testosterone levels, although it doesn't have as great of an effect on men who are already getting enough zinc in their body through their diet.

One of the most profound studies conducted between the relationship of zinc and testosterone levels was conducted in 1996. The difference between this study and others is that instead of giving the participants more of the mineral in question, this study actually fed young men a diet purposefully low in zinc so that they developed a zinc deficiency.

The researchers wanted to see how that zinc deficiency affected testosterone. The researchers tested the participants' testosterone levels before the study and then again after 20 weeks of the diet that was low in zinc. What they found was that the participants had a significant 75 percent decrease in testosterone levels when they consumed a low-zinc diet.

To cover all the bases of the relationship between zinc and testosterone levels, the same study took a look at elderly men, the part of the population that most often is associated with low testosterone levels. This is because of the fact that testosterone levels in men begin dropping naturally every year at age 30, with a potential 1 percent reduction in testosterone levels each year.

The researchers of the study gave these elderly men a daily zinc supplement. And what they found was that the zinc supplement more than doubled the testosterone levels in the participants.

Plenty of other studies abound about the correlation between zinc and testosterone. A 2009 study looked at rats, treating them with 5 milligrams per day of a zinc supplement. The results? The rats who received this treatment were proven to have better sexual function.

What the overall research has found is that the male body needs more zinc than the female body, and that having enough zinc in the body is essential not just for the production of testosterone, but for the release of it as well, so that the testosterone that is actually being produced by the body is being put to use effectively. The same is true of zinc's effect on athletic performance hormones, growth hormone and insulin-like growth factor-1.

So why does it work this way? It's because of the chemical processes that zinc is a vital part of that results in either producing testosterone or making it effective. Studies have shown that low zinc levels can lead to an increase in estrogen receptors and a decrease in androgen receptors, of which testosterone is a part. Zinc helps the body convert androstenedione into testosterone, an essential part in the creation process. And, much like vitamin D, low zinc levels may possibly increase aromatization of testosterone to estrogen.

The fact is that the male prostate tissue requires 10 times more zinc than other cells in the body to stay healthy. And if the body is low on zinc, the body is more susceptible to prostate cancer, as the body then has trouble accumulating zinc and fighting off the cancerous cells.

So how do you get more zinc?

Now that we know how important zinc is for not only testosterone levels in men but also for overall health, how much does a man need and how do they get it? Doctors say that adult men need about 11 milligrams of zinc per day in their diet. If you have low testosterone levels, you can seek to increase that amount to closer to 20 milligrams per day. Just be careful not to take any levels of zinc that can approach 40 milligrams per day, because that can cause toxicity in your body.

Zinc is actually found naturally in a lot of foods. The best sources of zinc are beans, meats, nuts, fish and other seafood. The best specific sources are raw oysters from the Pacific, beef lean chuck roast, baked beans, King Alaskan crab, lean ground beef, cooked lobster, lean pork loin, wild rice, green peas and plain yogurt. Vegetarians and vegans might have a lower level of zinc in their diet because of the foods they eat, so it's especially important that they make sure their levels are adequate in other ways.

There are plenty of zinc supplements on the market, and they are all good to take if you have a zinc deficiency, or a testosterone deficiency. The first step to find out whether you need more zinc is to have your blood tested for both zinc levels and testosterone levels. You need to get them both tested because you might need more zinc if you have a zinc deficiency; however, you might also need more zinc even if you're not deficient if you have low testosterone.

As always, the best way to get any vitamin and mineral into your body is through a diet that contains a high level of that vitamin or mineral. Consuming our nutrients through our food is the most effective way of getting the proper nutrients on a daily basis. If that's not possible for you, though, a zinc supplement is recommended.

They key with zinc supplements, as with any, is to read the labels to find out how much zinc you'll be getting by taking it, and compare that to the current zinc levels in your body. Most adult men daily multi-vitamins contain some level of zinc. That may be enough for your specific body or it may not.

If the multi-vitamin route isn't sufficient for you, then you can certainly take a zinc supplement. Remember, while adult males need more zinc than women and having extra zinc will help our immune system and testosterone levels, you don't want to have too much zinc in your body.

Too high levels can actually be toxic to your body and do way worse damage than low levels of zinc. In fact, too much zinc in your body can do the exact opposite to your immune system than its benefits – it can cause fever, cough, nausea, cholesterol changes, mineral imbalances and overall reduced immune function.

Therefore, doctors recommend that if you're taking a zinc-only supplement, you take one with a relatively low dose, around 8 milligrams to 12 milligrams per day. That's because you're most likely getting at least a little bit of zinc in your everyday diet, even if you're not purposefully doing so.

Doctors also recommend that if you take a zinc supplement you take an oral medication. There are zinc nasal sprays on the market, but studies have shown that these sprays have been linked to causing permanent taste and smell abnormalities, which is never a good thing. There are also zinc lozenges on the market, but some doctors say it can also alter your sense of smell for a few days.

You also need to be careful when taking zinc supplements based on other pills you may be taking. Zinc may interact with antibiotic medications and counteract the effects of it. So even though increasing your levels of zinc at the on-set of an infection could help stunt the spread of your disease or illness, once you start taking antibiotics for the infection, it's a good idea to refrain from taking your zinc supplement, or at least not taking as much.

Zinc supplements can also potentially cause an upset stomach or irritate the mouth. So, like any medication or supplement you take or intend to take, make sure to consult a doctor throughout the entire process.

Before diving into a high-zinc diet or taking a zinc supplement, have the levels of zinc and testosterone in your blood tested. It's an easy, painless blood test that will give you an overall picture of your body. Then, if you need more zinc in your body, that doctor can recommend a plan of action either through a zinc-focused diet and/or a daily multi-vitamin or zinc supplement. And, as always, if you experience any side effects or don't feel right on the new diet or supplement, consult your doctor again to figure out what may be going on.

Whatever your deficiency, whatever the reason you may need more zinc and however you go about doing it, know that zinc is one of the most essential nutrients our body needs for immune system function and specifically for healthy levels and function of testosterone in adult men.

THE ROLE OF MAGNESIUM & THE CORRECTION OF MICRONUTRIENT DEFICIENCIES LIKE SELENIUM IN INCREASING TESTOSTERONE PRODUCTION

Magnesium is another one of those essential nutrients that our body needs every day to function properly. It's one of those elements that we all learned on the periodic table when we were in school, but most of us have no practical knowledge about what it is and what it actually does.

Magnesium serves a plethora of functions for our body. In fact, scientists believe that magnesium plays a role in more than 300 biochemical reactions in the body. That's quite a lot.

Magnesium helps to maintain normal nerve and muscle function, keeps the heart beating at a steady pace, helps our bones remain strong and supports a healthy immune system. It also plays a role in regulating blood glucose levels and helps the production of energy and protein. Magnesium is also a defender, helping to prevent and manage high blood pressure, heart disease and diabetes, among other disorders.

There is also evidence that as an important micronutrient, magnesium plays a vital role in boosting testosterone in men, because it has an overall positive effect on anabolic hormonal status.

Magnesium is a tricky mineral, though. It's in a lot of the foods we eat, or at least the foods that are available for us to eat. There are supplements available to boost your magnesium levels should you have a deficiency, of course, but unlike some other vitamins and minerals, it's very important to pay attention to how much you're taking, because too much magnesium can be fatal.

That said, magnesium is important enough that ensuring you have a healthy level of it in your body is essential for basic bodily functions. And for those who have low levels of magnesium, or low levels of testosterone, a switch to a magnesium-rich diet or adding a magnesium supplement could prove very beneficial.

What is magnesium and what does it do?

Magnesium belongs to the family of electrolytes, which means it's a mineral that carries an electric charge when it is dissolved in the blood and other body fluids. When most people think of electrolytes, they think of those essential nutrients that your body needs after a good workout to help your body recover. They're touted as one of the huge benefits of popular replenishing sports drinks.

Not surprisingly, then, researchers have found that when you are exercising, you may need 10 percent to 20 percent more magnesium than when you're resting. That's magnesium acting as an electrolyte at its best – moving blood sugar into your muscles and disposing of lactic acid. Other studies have shown that magnesium supplements can also boost exercise performance in athletes.

Most of the magnesium that is found in the human body, though, is uncharged. Instead, most of the magnesium in our bodies is either bound to proteins or stored in our bones – where more than half our body's magnesium lives. This fact just further goes to show how important magnesium is for our bones and our body's structure.

Magnesium is very much needed to build bone and teeth strength as well as normal nerve and muscle function. Magnesium also plays a crucial role in metabolism of calcium and of potassium in the body. Basically, it serves in a multi-function capacity, chipping in here and there where it's needed.

Magnesium helps maintain healthy brain function, maintains a healthy heartbeat, helps regulate muscle contractions, may lower blood pressure, may reduce the risk of heart disease, may improve blood sugar control in Type 2 diabetes, can improve your sleep quality, may help combat migraines and may help reduce symptoms of depression. That's quite a lot of roles to play!

Since magnesium has so many purposes, our body needs a lot of it to function properly – at least a lot compared to other minerals. In fact, magnesium is the fourth most abundant mineral in the human body. Adult males need about 400 to 420 milligrams per day of magnesium, while adult women need about 310 to 320 milligrams per day.

If you have a diet that is high in protein, calcium or vitamin D, your body may require even more magnesium than the daily recommended intake. As always, consult with your doctor and/or a nutritionist to see exactly what your particular body may require.

Unfortunately, just because it is important doesn't mean that everyone is getting enough of it. A recent study found that 68 percent of American adults aren't meeting the daily recommended intake of magnesium. And similar statistics abound for other developed countries like the United States.

Not having enough magnesium in your body can lead to elevated inflammation markers. This, then, can make you susceptible to heart disease, diabetes, osteoporosis and some forms of cancer.

Where is magnesium found and why don't we have enough of it?

Magnesium is found naturally in a lot of foods that are available to us. As with nutrient's, reaching the daily recommended intake of magnesium is best to do primarily through eating whole foods. While taking a supplement can be a good way to get the job done, and may even be necessary for some, the most effective and healthy way to feed your body is by eating healthy foods.

A quarter-cup (or 16 grams) of pumpkin seeds contain 46 percent of the recommended daily intake for adult men. A cup of boiled spinach (39 percent), boiled Swiss chard (38 percent), cooked black beans (30 percent), flaxseeds (27 percent) or boiled beat greens (24 percent) are also excellent sources of magnesium.

Coming in next on the list of magnesium-rich foods are one ounce of almonds (20 percent), cashews (20 percent) or dark chocolate (16 percent); one medium avocado (15 percent); and 3.5 ounces of tofu (13 percent) or salmon (9 percent).

If you look over the list of magnesium-rich foods above, you can see why it's not hard to imagine that a lot of people – most, actually – consume a diet that's magnesium deficient.

The changing dietary habit of people around the developed world is a major reason for this. How many of us are consistently consuming a diet loaded with pumpkin seeds, black beans, almonds, tofu and even spinach? The answer is probably not a lot of us.

We live in an ever-changing global society today where people are busier than ever. The days of preparing a fresh-cooked homemade meal every night have gone by the wayside, or have at least reduced in number, replaced with meals that are store bought or eaten out.

Other factors are also in play for why so many people are magnesium deficient. Over the last 70 years, the way our food is grown and then processed has had a significant impact on the level of magnesium in our foods. Industrialized agriculture around the world has contributed to the diminishing amounts of magnesium in our foods. Some of the ways in which farmers and agricultural businesses processes food in order to preserve its shelf life and ship it around the world have actually removed a good amount of the natural magnesium in these products. In addition, the soil quality has been compromised from what we're putting into it, and because of the state of the environment as a whole.

Dr. Mildred Seeling laid out the issue quite plainly in her book "The Magnesium Factor." In it, she wrote, "if restaurant, homemade, or store-bought food contains fat, refined flour, and/or sugar as one or more of the major ingredients, it is a low-magnesium, and quite possibly a high-calorie, food. A steady diet of such foods, year after year, can produce magnesium deficit and, with it, metabolic syndrome X – a major factor in heart disease."

What this means is that the way in which we are consuming

our meals today is one of the biggest contributing factors to why a lot of us have a magnesium deficiency. And even if we are consciously eating magnesium-rich foods, we still might not be getting enough magnesium in our diets because of the way our foods are grown and processed nowadays. This is why more and more people are relying on magnesium supplements to attain healthy levels of the mineral.

Magnesium and testosterone

Magnesium has been found to be positively associated with total testosterone. Maybe it shouldn't be a surprise, then, that more and more adult males are faced with testosterone deficiencies. While magnesium isn't the only factor in a person's testosterone levels, the fact that it is at least a major contributing factor could be an answer as to why low-T levels are on the rise. Since most adult males aren't getting nearly enough magnesium into their bodies, should we be surprised that the number of adult males with low testosterone levels is increasing as well?

Magnesium's role in this case is to increase the bioavailability of testosterone. As we've discussed a few times before, as men age, sex hormone binding globulin (SHBG) concentrations increase. The SHBG binds to testosterone, making it unavailable for the body to use. This is not a good thing, obviously.

What magnesium does is it attracts testosterone to it. So when there are adequate, or increasing, levels of magnesium in your body, the testosterone that is there binds with it instead of the SHBG. This, then, keeps the testosterone "free," which keeps it available for use, thereby increasing its anabolic effects. It's pretty simple, actually.

A recent study looked at young males between the ages of 18 and 22. The researchers gave the participants of the study an additional 10 milligrams of magnesium per kilogram of body weight per day. That's a whole lot of extra magnesium, to be sure. For a 220-pound person, that would equate to one gram, or 1,000 milligrams, which is more than double the daily recommended intake.

For the purposes of the study, though, the results were quite staggering.

After taking this daily supplement for only four weeks, the researchers found that the participants tested at higher levels for both free and total testosterone levels. And when the participants were doing exercises or other similar strenuous activities, they had an even greater increase in testosterone levels. While taking that much magnesium on a consistent basis over a long period of time definitely isn't recommended, the study did accomplish what it sought to do – make the solid connection that magnesium is a solid factor in testosterone production and utilization.

There are some drawbacks from the above-referenced study, however. Sure, the effects of magnesium supplementation are quite eye opening, but who in their right mind would take that much magnesium per day, on top of everything they are eating in their diets? Not only is that not realistic, it's not healthy, either.

So let's look at a second study and see what its effects were. For this study, the men who participated were between the ages of 18 and 30. They were split into two groups, with one group given a daily total of eight milligrams per kilogram of weight of magnesium. The other group was given a placebo to measure the results against. This dosage included what they were consuming in their diet, though, so that the total amount of magnesium they consumed – both through food and through a supplement – was eight milligrams per kilogram of weight. That's a little more realistic.

The participants of this study consumed that amount of magnesium over a seven-week period, and they were asked to do a mild amount of exercise three times per week. This "mild" exercise was only doing three sets of 10 reps for leg extensions and leg presses, so not a strenuous workout to say the least.

What the researchers found was that both groups in the study gained strength over the length of the study. But the group that was on the magnesium-controlled plan gained substantially more, leading the researchers to conclude that magnesium plays a positive role in protein synthesis at the ribosomal level.

But what does this have to do with testosterone? Well, an improvement in protein synthesis will in an indirect way allow your body to produce more testosterone, and it will allow the testosterone in your body to operate more freely and, therefore, be more effective in what it's supposed to do.

We can also relate this back to something we hit on just a minute ago. Guess what happens when a person lacks protein in their diet? Well, it starts secreting more of the sex hormone binding globulin (SHBG)! Pretty amazing, isn't it?

So let's break this equation down then. Magnesium plays a positive role in protein synthesis at the ribosomal level. When there is enough protein in the body, and when there is enough magnesium in the body to help process that protein, the body doesn't produce as much SHBG. And with less SHBG in the body to bind to it, the testosterone that is in the body is able to instead remain free and bind to magnesium instead. It's a pretty fascinating cycle.

A third recent study looked at men over the age of 65 – a group that is very commonly associated with low testosterone levels, due in large part to the fact that our bodies can lose up to 1 percent of testosterone levels each year naturally, starting at the age of 30. What the study found was that men in the study group who had higher levels of magnesium also had higher levels of both free testosterone and total testosterone.

This study didn't conclusively find that the magnesium in the blood actually caused the higher levels of testosterone in these same men. However, combining the results of this study with the results of other studies that tackled the same subject could draw a distinct line between the role of magnesium in testosterone levels and effectiveness.

Selenium and testosterone

Selenium is a lot like magnesium, and as such, it has similar effects on testosterone levels. Selenium is a trace mineral in the body that is found in many proteins.

Certain forms of selenium act as antioxidants, fighting free radicals that are in the body. This process ends up fighting off what could be major damage to the body's cells, which ultimately could lead to some serious disease and illness. In this role as an antioxidant, selenium helps reduce oxidative stress and cell damage.

While selenium has important roles in the body that have to do with cells, lowering blood pressure and preventing some bad things from happening, it has also been found to boost testosterone levels slightly and also have a positive effect on male reproductive health.

A study in The Journal or Urology found that infertile males who took a supplement of only 200 micrograms of selenium a day for 26 weeks saw a slight increase in their testosterone levels.

Selenium has also been found to increase sperm count and sperm quality. While selenium may not be a huge booster when it comes to significantly increasing testosterone, it does play a crucial role in testosterone formation and creating quality sperm. In a 2009 study, 468 men were given selenium for 26 weeks, and the results found that these men had enhanced semen quality and elevated serum testosterone.

Selenium has also been found to prevent against prostate cancer, which is connected to overall male sexual health. It's able to do this due to its antioxidant properties, helping your body to minimize cell damage that is often linked to prostate cancer. People who have a selenium deficiency are at a higher risk for prostate cancer than those who do not.

Unlike some other nutrients we've discussed, your body doesn't need a lot of selenium at all on a daily basis. In fact, the recommended daily intake is just 55 micrograms per day for adult males.

Selenium is found most prominently in seafoods and organ meats, but can also be found in muscle meats, cereals and grains, and dairy products. The most selenium-rich foods include Brazil nuts, yellowfin tuna, halibut, sardines, ham, shrimp, beef steak, turkey, beef liver, chicken, cottage cheese, brown rice, ground beef and eggs.

Other micronutrients and testosterone

Throughout this chapter, we've dealt specifically with the health benefits and testosterone-boosting nature of magnesium. In past articles, we also talked about similar benefits of other micronutrients such as zinc and vitamin D.

The research is pretty clear: Micronutrients play an extremely critical role in testosterone production, testosterone health and testosterone utilization, in addition to being essential for other functions in the body. A lot of this discovery has been found through research conducted more recently, over the last 15 years or so. That's why in the supplement marketplace, you're seeing a shift from what was the original testosterone- or libido-boosting supplements to the focus now on supplements focused on at least one of these micronutrients.

Those old testosterone supplements were mainly just a bunch of herbs, and maybe even spices, that were touted to increase a man's sex drive. But as we've discussed quite clearly, testosterone isn't all about having a better sex drive. That is certainly one of the things that decreases as men age and/or in men who have a low level of testosterone, but it isn't nearly the only role that testosterone plays.

Having low levels of testosterone can be dangerous, especially for men, because it can be associated with thinner bones, weight gain, lower energy and feelings of depression. So having adequate levels of testosterone really is essential for any person, but especially for adult males who tend to experience a regular drop in testosterone levels as they age.

That's why more and more people are focusing on proper nutrition when it comes to the three most important micronutrients for testosterone levels – magnesium, zinc and vitamin D. Each of these micronutrients plays an important role, either directly or indirectly, in supporting healthy and adequate production of testosterone and in keeping as much testosterone in the body free as possible, preventing it from binding with things such as SHBG. There has even been a direct link found between not only these micronutrients and testosterone, but also each of these nutrients separately with each other.

By addressing a micronutrient deficiency, you are not only addressing the potential issue of having low testosterone levels, but you are taking care of your overall health as well. It's no secret that magnesium, zinc and vitamin D all play important roles in many different functions throughout your body. It's also no surprise that many people with low testosterone levels are also found to be deficient in magnesium, zinc and vitamin D.

The problem isn't that we aren't sure if we need adequate levels of these micronutrients in our body. The challenge, instead, is that none of these three micronutrients are readily found in foods that we eat every day. Sure, there foods that are high in magnesium, high in zinc or high in vitamin D, and there are even some foods that are high in all three. But it's harder to get these nutrients naturally than it is to, say, get an adequate amount of protein or to limit the amount of sugar and carbohydrates you eat.

The first step in making sure you have an adequate amount of micronutrients in your body is to consult with a doctor and have him or her test your levels of testosterone, magnesium, zinc and vitamin D. Then, once you have a clear picture of where your deficiencies lie, then you can create a plan with both your doctor and maybe even a nutritionist around how to get enough of these micronutrients in your body.

That nutrition plan is step two in the process. This may include eating more leafy greens, more beans, more nuts and even some fish. Step three in the process is supplementing your diet with pills for magnesium, zinc and vitamin D separately – depending on what your deficiency is – or taking a daily adult men's multi-vitamin that contains a sufficient amount of each for your body.

The final step is important as well – you need to get enough exercise. Living a healthy lifestyle isn't just about what you put into your body, but also how you treat it in terms of your activity level. And when it comes to adequate testosterone levels and healthy testosterone functions, it's imperative that you are exercising every week as well.

HOW THE AMINO ACID GLYCINE & L-THEANINE SIGNAL TO YOUR BODY TO PRODUCE HIGHER T BY TRIGGERING LH PRODUCTION

W e've talked a lot about how you can boost testosterone levels naturally by incorporating essential nutrients and micronutrients into your diet, or by taking supplements of these nutrients and micronutrients to give you the results you are looking for. However, what we've discussed thus far has dealt mainly with minerals and vitamins that most people are familiar with – zinc, magnesium, vitamin D and even boron and selenium.

What we haven't discussed yet, though, are amino acids. Most people are familiar with the term amino acid, but many people probably don't have an intricate understanding of exactly what amino acids do. Sure, most of us know that amino acids are in some way associated with proteins, so it's easy for us to deduce that amino acids play a role in the things that proteins do – things such as building muscle and providing health energy.

But that's not all that amino acids do. While amino acids are considered the "building blocks" of proteins, they're also needed to help build proteins and synthesize hormones and neurotransmitters. As such, some people take amino acid supplements to do things such as boost athletic performance and even improve mood.

There are 20 different amino acids in total, and while only nine of them are classified as "essential," because they can't be produced by your body naturally and must be obtained through your diet, all amino acids play a vital role in your body's health.

What do amino acids do?

As we mentioned, amino acids play a vital role in building protein in the body, but they are also essential for other functions in your body. While each of the 20 amino acids play a slightly different role, or, rather, have a slightly different specialty, they all have very similar benefits.

Generally speaking, amino acids can help improve your mood and, as a byproduct, your sleep habits. That's because amino acids help produce serotonin, a chemical that regulates mood, sleep and behaviors. Low serotonin levels have been associated with depression and sleep disturbances, so having a healthy level of it is key for your body to stay even-keeled and get enough rest.

Amino acids also serve an essential role in three areas that are associated with testosterone – boosting exercise performance, preventing muscle loss and promoting weight loss. Amino acids help to alleviate fatigue, improve athletic performance and even stimulate muscle recovery after exercise. They also help prevent muscle breakdown and preserve lean body mass. And, finally, amino acids naturally also help to reduce body fat percentage.

While none of those characteristics of amino acids draws a direct line to testosterone production, we are beginning to see similarities to the benefits of both.

What is glycine?

Glycine is one of the 20 amino acids, but probably one that you've never heard of. That's because it's not classified as an essential amino acid. Further, glycine is the second most abundant amino acid in the human body, so in the world of amino acids, it's not one that we'd tend to think needs to be focused on.

However, studies have shown that despite it being one of the most abundant amino acids in our body, plenty of people don't get enough of it nowadays, and that could have a serious negative effect on testosterone levels, especially in older men.

Glycine levels never used to be a problem, and for some parts of the world, it probably still isn't. So what has changed? The eating habits of most people today have changed dramatically, and that has had a significant effect on how much glycine most of us are consuming.

But it's not exactly what you are thinking. We aren't getting lower levels of glycine in our diet because we're eating more unhealthy foods now than we collectively did in the past. Instead, we're getting less glycine because most of us don't subscribe to the practice of eating the whole animal.

You see, glycine is found most abundantly in animal tissue, which are parts of an animal's body that we don't often eat anymore. Glycine is found in the skin, bones, ligaments and tendons of animals. What we consume, mainly, are animal muscles, which don't contain glycine. So, as a result, we as a collective people aren't getting the same amount of glycine today as we once did when eating the entire animal wasn't a choice but a necessity.

Not surprisingly, glycine helps the areas of our body that it helps in animals. It helps us build strong ligaments, tendons and healthy skin. It also plays a big role in brain health. Studies have shown that taking glycine before bed can result in deeper, more restful sleep. And getting good sleep is one of the most important things our body needs. In fact, poor sleep has been proven, among other things, to reduce testosterone levels.

Glycine has also been shown to boost growth hormone levels substantially. And, finally, glycine has been found to bind with certain toxins in your body, which allows them to be released from your body in a safe way, and preventing these toxins from binding with other things in your body, such as testosterone.

You can increase the amount of glycine in your body by simply eating more collagen, which is found non-muscle meats and gelatin, but it can also be obtained through a supplement. Glycine supplements are desirable, too. Because they have a sweet taste, they can be simply added to teas, coffees or any other beverage as a replacement for sugar.

What is L-theanine?

L-theanine is an amino acid that, not surprisingly, doesn't get a lot of publicity. It's even hard to say. But it's an amino acid that some people in the world get a lot of, while others hardly get any at all. That's because it is found most abundantly in one product – tea leaves.

L-Theanine belongs to the amino acid group of glutamine. Like glycine, it is classified as a non-essential amino acid, but that doesn't mean it's not important for the body.

Because it's found naturally in tea leaves, it's not hard to draw the conclusion that L-theanine has been proven to promote relaxation without drowsiness. Just think about the well-known effects of tea. It's a low-caffeine beverage that helps the mind and body relax. The reason for that? It's the L-theanine that's contained inside the tea leaves. The powerful amino acid is what plays a role in anxiety and stress relief, benefits that are widely associated with drinking a nice, relaxing cup of tea, especially before bed at night.

Other benefits of L-theanine are that it helps increase focus, leads to better immunity, helps prevent tumors and treat cancer, keeps your blood pressure under control, improves your sleep – which has an ever-important role in preventing low testosterone levels – and helps relieve sinusitis.

L-theanine is also extremely powerful because it has antioxidant properties. Antioxidants, as we discussed before, fight free radicals in the body. By helping to rid the body of harmful toxins, antioxidants play a vital role in fighting against disease and illness, and in helping the body perform its normal, necessary functions such as producing, releasing and utilizing testosterone.

L-theanine has also been shown to regulate arousal, both sexual and non-sexual, in the brain as well as help with weight loss – two characteristics also associated with healthy testosterone.

L-theanine also plays a pivotal role in the release of dopamine in your body. This, then, results in higher levels of testosterone directly, and also a more effective production and usage of the testosterone as L-theanine helps keep the body healthy overall by regulating healthy sleep habits.

If you aren't getting enough L-theanine in your diet naturally, it's easy to get more. Green tea is especially high in the amino acid, and it can be consumed either as a traditional hot tea or as an iced tea. You can even get two essential amino acids in your body at once if you steep a nice cup of green tea and then add a glycine supplement to it as a sweetener.

If you don't like to drink tea at all – whether in a hot or cold form – you can also buy chewable L-theanine tablets to take as a supplement. Doctors recommend that taking anywhere from 50 milligrams to 200 milligrams a day of L-theanine is what will have the best results for your body. As always, consult with a doctor and nutritionist to find out how much specifically you should take, which they will determine based on your current levels of L-theanine and the specific reasons you need to increase your levels of it.

What is luteinizing hormone?

Luteinizing hormone is better known to most people as its acronym, LH. Those of us that are familiar with LH, or at least have a base knowledge of the name and maybe what it does, are used to hearing it associated more with women. That's because LH plays a very important role in ovulation. A surge in LH once a month is the trigger that causes the ovary to release the egg.

Men might be most familiar with LH if they are trying to conceive a child with their wife and might be having at least some difficulty doing so. That's because in these instances, a woman will often measure her LH levels because it's an indicator of when her fertile window will occur that month. Ovulation is obviously necessary for conception, and LH surge is necessary for the release of the egg (or ovulation), and therefore, a rise in LH level would indicate that ovulation has occurred or is going to occur.

Other than playing an important role in conception in a woman's body, though, what does LH have to do with men? A lot, actually. LH is one of the best predictors of overall testicular function, and is a key hormone that can help in the evaluation of male fertility.

LH does this by commanding the Leydig Cells in the testicle

to produce testosterone. If there is no LH in the testicles, then the Leydig Cells don't produce testosterone. If there is LH present, then testosterone is produced. So it seems, then, that there is no more important thing than LH when it comes to testosterone production. If there is no LH, there is no testosterone. Lower levels of LH, similarly, will result in lower levels of testosterone.

The thinking would be that those of us who have lower levels of testosterone and are suffering from a testosterone deficiency can focus on LH levels, and it will solve all our problems. That's not necessarily true, directly but it's a great place to start.

The human body is truly an amazing thing. The adult male body can sense that testosterone levels are chronically low, and in these cases, the brain responds by increasing the production of LH to help stimulate the production of testosterone. Similarly, if testosterone levels are too high, the brain can decide to produce less LH.

That sounds all fine and dandy, but those of us with low levels of testosterone might respond by asking, "What gives? If the brain will naturally react to chronically low levels of testosterone by producing more LH, why do I still have a testosterone deficiency?"

Those are good questions, of course. The answer is not so simple. When testosterone levels are low, the body will respond by making sure it produces normal levels of LH, but normal levels of LH might not be enough for your body to produce enough of that extra testosterone you may need. That means it's possible that you could have low testosterone levels but normal LH levels. It's also possible, in some cases, for adult men to have high levels of LH but low levels of testosterone.

No matter what your specific situation in terms of levels of LH and testosterone, there is no denying the cause-and-effect relationship between LH and testosterone production. At its purest, chemical foundation, LH directly causes the production of testosterone, so LH is an essential hormone in and of itself for overall adult male health.

Like anything, it's important to get your levels of LH tested by a doctor before you make any decisions to focus on increasing your levels of it. Since LH is a hormone, it's easy to get tested for it. In fact, doctors can order a blood test that can measure your entire panel of hormones, which will include both LH and testosterone, giving you a clearer overall picture of your hormonal health.

Healthy ranges of LH in an adult male are between 2.0 mIU/mL and 9.0 mIU/mL. Levels that are lower than 1.0 or higher than 10.0 are usually an indication that there is a problem somewhere.

Just looking at LH levels does not give you the perfect snapshot of what might be the problem if you have low testosterone levels. If LH levels are high, for example, it's still possible to have low testosterone levels. This situation could indicate that there is damage to either the testicle or the pituitary gland that is preventing all this extra LH from producing adequate levels of testosterone.

Generally speaking, though, elevated levels of LH will result in elevated levels of testosterone, as long as there is no other damage or defect in your body. Some of the reasons you may be experiencing low LH levels are genetic conditions such as Kallman's Syndrome, both cancerous and benign pituitary tumors, head trauma, and auto-immune disorders.

In addition, studies have shown that men who take external

androgens such as testosterone-boosting products, anabolic steroids and other performance enhancers can actually result in lower LH levels. That's because these androgens trick the brain into thinking the body is naturally producing high levels of testosterone, so the brain thinks it also has enough LH in the system, and therefore, it slows down the production of LH.

That's an interesting revelation – that these external androgens, which were once the go-to for men who wanted to boost their testosterone, can actually have a negative effect on their body's testosterone production. It's yet another reason why boosting your testosterone through natural means is much better for your body overall.

What does glycine and L-theanine have to do with LH?

We now know the importance of glycine and L-theanine and LH in the body, especially the essential roles they all play in overall male health and specifically in relation to testosterone. But what do the amino acids glycine and L-theanine have to do with LH?

Studies have shown that these non-essential amino acids, and all amino acids in general, play a vital role in the release and synthesis of LH and testosterone in humans. Think of it in terms of this cause-and-effect relationship:

<u>Healthy levels of the amino acids glycine and L-theanine trigger the production of LH</u>; healthy levels of LH triggers the production of testosterone; so, therefore, healthy levels of the amino acids glycine and L-theanine are essential for your body to produce healthy levels of testosterone.

The question becomes, then, does increasing the levels of glycine and L-theanine in your body have a direct causal result of having increased levels of testosterone? The answer is yes.

A recent study took a look at just this question, investigating the effect of amino acids on the release of LH and also the release of testosterone in the serum of both humans and rats.

In the human aspect of the research, the study gave a group of 23 men a daily dose of amino acids for 12 days and gave another group of 20 men a placebo to serve as a measuring stick. What the study found was that the amino acid "increases the release and synthesis of LH through the involvement of cGMP as a second messenger" in humans.

The study's conclusion, therefore, was rather straightforward: The amino acid occurs "principally in the pituitary gland and testes and has a role in the regulation of the release and synthesis of LH and testosterone in humans and rats."

This study just goes to prove that having proper levels of amino acids such as glycine and L-theanine in the body can result in higher levels of testosterone because the amino acids play a direct role in the production and release of LH, which is directly responsible for producing testosterone.

How do you get more glycine and L-theanine?

We've already discussed the main sources of glycine and L-theanine that you can consume as part of your regular diet. It might be difficult – or, rather, not pleasing – for most people to get more glycine in their diet. That's because glycine is found most predominantly in parts of animals that most people throw away: the skin, bones, connective tissues, tendons and ligaments.

Just because a food is high in protein does not mean that it will be high in glycine. Meat and dairy products do contain some glycine, but not a lot, and probably not enough if you're looking to increase your intake of it as a way to boost your testosterone.

You can get increased levels of glycine into your diet by making bone broth or by incorporating gelatin into some of the meals you make, because both products contain collagen. Some levels of glycine are also found in beans, spinach, kale, cabbage, banana and kiwi.

L-theanine is a little easier to incorporate into your diet. That's because L-theanine is found naturally in tea leaves, which for modern people is probably more pleasing on the taste buds than animal connective tissues or bone broth. If you like the taste of hot or iced tea, especially green tea, then it can be very easy to get an increased amount of both glycine and L-theanine into your body. This can be done by dissolving a glycine supplement – which can act as a sugar substitute because of its sweet taste – into a cup of tea.

If you don't like tea, though, you don't have to fret. Both glycine and L-theanine can be found in supplement form, so you can make sure you get enough of both in your body. Even though glycine and L-theanine are classified as non-essential amino acids, they have been proven to be essential in the production of testosterone because of the effects that they have on the production of LH.

LOWERING CORTISOL & REGULATING ESTROGEN WITH KSM-66 ASHWAGANDHA CAN INCREASE YOUR T-LEVELS & THE EGG MYTH? HOW HIGHER CHOLESTEROL INTAKE CAN INCREASE YOUR TESTOSTERONE

Ashwagandha is an ancient Indian herb that has been used for centuries in the large Asian nation. Like many things in this world, it is hard to imagine the first person who discovered ashwagandha and decided that it would be a good idea to try to process and consume it. The reason we say this is because in Sanskrit, the word ashwagandha means "odor of the horse."

The reason it was named that is because the smell of the herb's root apparently resembled the odor of a sweaty horse. That doesn't sound too pleasant. And it certainly doesn't sound like something most people would smell and then decide to consume.

However, we should all be thankful that that first person who discovered ashwagandha did, and that he or she decided to take his or her discovery one step further to realize the wonders of the root he or she found.

You see, ashwagandha is quite the powerful herb. It is sometimes referred to as "Indian ginseng," because ashwagandha is used in India in a very similar fashion to how people practicing traditional Chinese medicine use ginseng. As such, it is used to treat an extremely wide variety of diseases, illnesses and ailments in the human body.

Ashwagandha is so powerful and has so many benefits that it is beginning to find its way into the western world.

KSM-66 Ashwagandha is one of the most concentrated ashwagandha root extracts on the market today, and one of the most powerful and good-for-you supplements around. As we'll see in just a bit, the herb has various benefits to just about anyone, from reducing stress and lowering anxiety, to improving brain function and preventing disease, to increasing testosterone levels and improving fertility.

What is ashwagandha?

Ashwagandha is an Indian herb that comes from a plant in the nightshade family. It's a small shrub with yellow flowers that grows natively in India and North Africa. Other plants in this variety include tomatoes peppers, potatoes, pimentos and goji berries. It is often used in Ayurveda, a natural, alternative system of medicine that has been used for centuries in the Indian subcontinent. In that practice, ashwagandha is considered a "Rasayana herb," meaning it is an elixir that works not in a very specific way to heal the body but in a global way to improve health and longevity in humans. That designation means it has a wide variety of benefits, as we'll soon see.

At its base, ashwagandha is considered an adaptogen, meaning it is a nontoxic medication that "normalizes functions disturbed by chronic stress." That is to say it corrects hormone imbalances. This is the area for which ashwagandha is perhaps best known – its ability to reduce stress.

Ashwagandha has been proven to lower cortisol levels in

humans. Cortisol, which, as we've discussed before, is known as the "stress hormone." The adrenal glands release cortisol in response to stress or when your body's blood sugar levels get too low. Sometimes, though, cortisol levels become too elevated in the human body, which can lead to high blood sugar levels and increased fat storage in our belly.

The good news is that ashwagandha has been proven to reduce cortisol levels. One study in particular took a look at chronically stressed adults. These people were given a supplement of ashwagandha, and what the researchers found was that after a period of time taking the supplement, they saw a large decrease in cortisol levels. In fact, one of the groups in the study that took the highest dose of ashwagandha reported a decrease in cortisol levels of 30 percent.

The way ashwagandha works in this fashion is that it helps to block the "stress pathway" in the brain by regulating chemical signals in the nervous system. By lowering levels of cortisol and reducing overall stress, ashwagandha has been shown to help reduce anxiety and insomnia as well. This makes sense, of course, because stress is well-known to be a major cause of these and other ailments.

One 60-day study gave people with chronic stress a supplement of ashwagandha and found that those who took the supplement reported an average 69 percent drop in anxiety and insomnia. Similarly, another study reported an 88 percent reduction in anxiety after taking ashwagandha supplement for only six weeks.

Because of the regulation of cortisol and also the decrease in anxiety, ashwagandha has also been associated with helping to reduce the symptoms of depressions. When we are less stressed, and when we are less anxious, we often can feel less depressed, too. Yes, stress and anxiety don't necessarily cause depression – or even vice versa – but the three ailments can often occur all together inside one person. So ashwagandha, then, seems to hit the trifecta of emotional ailments, all by calming the body and reducing cortisol levels.

Ashwagandha has many other proven benefits as well. Some of these include the ability to improve brain function and memory, reduce inflammation, reduce blood sugar levels, induce fat cell death, fight infections, promote heart health and fight against cancer. All these reasons are why the ancient Indian medicinal practice considered it such a beneficial herb.

What is ashwagandha's relation to testosterone?

Among the benefits of ashwagandha is an increase in testosterone levels. This is done in both direct and indirect ways, as we'll soon see. Let's start with the direct ways.

Studies have shown that ashwagandha supplements are effective ways to increase testosterone levels and improve the overall reproductive health of adult males. One particular study looked at a group of 75 infertile men who were treated with ashwagandha. After the test period, these men were found to have increased sperm counts and motility, and they also showed an increased level of testosterone.

Taking ashwagandha is also a proven way to increase muscle mass and strength, which are key areas where testosterone also has a profound effect. Men who have taken daily ashwagandha supplements have been shown to gain muscle strength after only 30 days, while they also experience a reduction in body fat percentage at the same time.

Most of the ways in which ashwagandha has a positive effect on testosterone are through more indirect ways, though. This is to say that taking an ashwagandha supplement has been shown to be better for overall reproductive health not by boosting testosterone directly, but by boosting and supporting all the things that are important, and even essential, for having adequate levels of testosterone.

Perhaps the strongest way that ashwagandha has a positive effect on testosterone levels is because of its calming and relaxing effect on the body, which is done through the regulation and reduction of cortisol levels, as we discussed earlier. In essence, ashwagandha helps to balance hormones in the body. This, then, also improves overall fertility by promoting relaxation and decreasing stress.

The more relaxed and less stressed, anxious and depressed you are, the better your body functions overall. That's because a relaxed and worry-free body is one in which all the hormones are balanced and running in synch. Let's not forget that testosterone is a hormone, and a very important one at that. So when stress and anxiety are high, that causes hormone levels to be off. As a result, testosterone levels can often be lower in people who are not relaxed, stressed out and/or having feelings of anxiety and/or depression.

This has been proven to be true. High stress is directly associated with low testosterone.

A large study of just this effect was conducted at The University of Texas at Austin. It found that when cortisol levels increase in order to respond to high levels of stress, the body is "mobilized to escape danger," first and foremost. As a result, it is focused on that fight or flight mentality, and not on any factors that influence testosterone production.

What the study found, then, was that cortisol actually works in opposition to testosterone. When cortisol levels are high – which happens when the body and mind are experiencing a lot of stress – then testosterone levels are often low. This is why regulating cortisol to a normal level is so important to having healthy and normal levels of testosterone.

Robert Josephs, the lead researcher for the study, laid this cause-and-effect relationship out in plain English:

"It makes good adaptive sense that testosterone's behavioral influence during an emergency situation gets blocked because engaging in behaviors that are encouraged by testosterone, such as mating, competition and aggression, during an imminent survival situation could be fatal," said Josephs, a professor of psychology at The University of Texas at Austin. "On the other hand, fight or flight behaviors encouraged by cortisol become more likely during an emergency situation when cortisol levels are high. Thus, it makes sense that the hormonal axes that regulate testosterone levels and cortisol levels are antagonistic."

Basically, it's ultra-important for adult males to have normal, regulated levels of both cortisol and testosterone. When stress and anxiety levels are high, though, it's also very important that cortisol kicks into high gear to respond. That, unfortunately, will result in lower testosterone. So people who are constantly stressed out or anxious will oftentimes have higher levels of cortisol and lower levels of testosterone.

Ashwagandha also helps promote healthy male fertility and healthy hormone levels in a number of ways. In addition to directly boosting testosterone levels and increasing sperm count and sperm quality, it has also been found to improve the overall function of the thyroid gland, which is in part responsible for regulating reproductive hormones. It's also been known to treat males with hypogonadism, which, again, is the reduction or absence of hormone secretion and other physiological activity of the gonads – which, in males, is the testes, where testosterone is produced.

Taking ashwagandha supplements has also be found to have a positive effect on improving the weight of testes, and has been found to have the ability to counteract the formation of Reactive Oxygen Species in infertile men.

Finally, in one of the most direct "indirect" ways that ashwagandha promotes testosterone production is how it benefits Luteinizing hormone, something that is better known as LH. As we've discussed before, LH is perhaps the best predictor of overall testicular function. It's a key hormone that can help in the evaluation of male fertility. But how?

LH does this by commanding the Leydig Cells in the testicle to produce testosterone. If there is no LH in the testicles, then the Leydig Cells don't produce testosterone. If there is LH present, then testosterone is produced. So it seems, then, that there is no more important thing than LH when it comes to testosterone production. If there is no LH, there is no testosterone. Lower levels of LH, similarly, will result in lower levels of testosterone.

So, again, if LH is not present in the testes, then testosterone will not be produced. Further, then, if the levels of LH in your body are low, then most likely you will have low levels of LH. That's why having healthy levels of LH is so important – because it directly results in the level of testosterone in the body. Since ashwagandha has been proven to increase LH in males with low levels of it or low levels of testosterone, it is easy to see the positive effects it can have on testosterone in general.

The best way to get ashwagandha? KSM-66 Ashwagandha

We now know that ashwagandha is a great way to promote healthy levels of cortisol, which then results in healthy levels of testosterone, among other things. And we know ashwagandha has plenty of other benefits for the body, including many direct and indirect effects on testosterone. But how do we get it and how much should we take?

Ashwagandha is available as a supplement in many forms, but perhaps the best product available is KSM-66 Ashwagandha. That's because it's the most concentrated ashwagandha root extract available. The extract can be taken directly, or it can also be used as a complementary ingredient in other dietary supplements such as a tea or smoothie.

KSM-66 Ashwagandha can come in powder, capsules, tables, soft gels and even liquids as well. It's a great supplement to take because it is pretty neutral, and doesn't have a bitter taste. In fact, KSM-66 Ashwagandha has been found to be three times less biter compared to other ashwagandha extracts or powders.

KSM-66 Ashwagandha has been proven through studies as an effective way to reduce stress and anxiety as well as improve sperm count and sexual health in men. It also has been shown to enhance heart function and endurance during exercise and improve strength during weight training.

The daily recommended intake for ashwagandha is 3 grams to 6 grams of the dried root daily. However, studies have shown that the most effective way to get the best benefits from ashwagandha is to take it in powder form, after it has been ground and dried, like it is in KSM-66 Ashwagandha. In this form, it is recommended to take 300 milligrams to 500 milligrams daily for maximum health benefits.

What about eggs?

What do eggs have to do with testosterone? The answer to that very good question is quite a lot, actually. But how?

Testosterone is produced in the body by cholesterol. As most of us know, your body needs at least some level of cholesterol to function, and there is also what's known as good cholesterol and bad cholesterol. In this regard, cholesterol is something that is good for you.

Cholesterol gets a really bad rap most of the time. Most of us make the conscious choice on our own to reduce the amount of cholesterol in our diets, and a lot of us are even told to do so by our doctors after maybe a blood test reveals our levels of cholesterol are too high. And it's true – too much cholesterol is not a good thing, and can lead to some nasty end results such as clogged arteries.

However, our bodies do need some cholesterol to function, and plenty of very healthy foods that are high in protein also have some high levels of good cholesterol. Cholesterol comes from fat, and fat is needed to do a lot of very positive things in our body. It's just that we don't want too much of it.

A recent study looked at just this aspect of fat – its positive results. A group of men ate more than 100 grams of fat per day for two weeks. After doing so, the study found that these men had less of a certain hormone than others. That hormone is sex-hormone binding globulin, or SHBG.

As we've talked about before, SHBG is a nasty and unwanted thing, especially when it comes to testosterone. That's because SHBG binds to testosterone and prevents it from being free. And free testosterone is the only form of testosterone that is available for your body to use effectively. These men who focused on consuming the 100 grams of fat per day had higher levels of free testosterone as a result.

This is not to say that we should all run out and start eating fat-heavy foods to boost our testosterone. In fact, doing so will probably have an adverse effect on our testosterone as a whole as we all start becoming overweight. Instead, the proper thing to do is to focus on eating health fats, fats that contain healthy cholesterol that will help reduce the amount of SHBG in our bodies and, therefore, increase our levels of free testosterone.

One of the best ways to do this is to eat eggs. Eggs are a wonderful option for humans of all ages and gender, but especially for adult males who may be suffering from low testosterone levels. Eggs are something that should be incorporated into the everyday diet of these men, and can be done so in any meal of the day.

The important thing to note, though, is that in order to get the most "bang for your buck," you have to eat the entire egg. A lot of healthy eating plans and diets will tout the power and preference of eating just the egg whites. That's because they are a healthier option for your body if you are trying to lose weight because they are high in protein and low in cholesterol and, therefore, calories.

However, eating only the egg weights is not suggested for people who are trying to focus on improving their testosterone levels. That's because the egg yolks contain more nutrients that the egg whites. So for men who are looking to increase their testosterone levels, it is essential to eat the entire egg, yolk and all.

Egg yolks get perhaps the worst wrap of any food when it comes to cholesterol. But keep in mind that this type of cholesterol that is found in egg yolks is actually the good type when it comes to dealing with people with low testosterone levels.

Furthermore, egg yolks are a rich source of vitamin D. And as we've discussed before, vitamin D has a positive influence on testosterone levels as well. In fact, studies have shown that taking a daily supplement of vitamin D can result in an average increase in testosterone levels of 25.2 percent.

So while cholesterol in general and eggs in specific have gotten a bad wrap over the years when it comes to being healthy and losing weight, the positive effects both have on testosterone levels outweigh the negatives for the men suffering from low T.

INTERMITTENT FASTING AS A LONG-TERM WAY OF BOOSTING YOUR TESTOSTERONE & EXTENDING YOUR LIFE

D o you want to lose weight? If you do, the solution is simple – just stop eating. That will make you lose weight.

Of course, we are not serious when we suggest that you stop eating altogether, no matter how overweight, unhealthy or unhappy with your body you are. Not eating is, well, a bad idea. Your body needs nutrients, it needs energy, to function throughout the day, and the only way to do that is to consume food.

Eating healthier, living an overall better lifestyle, is something we should all strive to do. Even the healthiest of people out there could probably use a little kick in the pants every once in a while when it comes to their eating habits.

In today's world, it has become too easy to not eat healthy, and many of us flock toward quick and easy food that is often loaded with stuff that is not good for our bodies. This has caused obesity to rise in the developed world almost world-wide, and it has resulted in higher rates of diabetes, lower testosterone levels in men and other diseases as well.

There are diet and weight-loss fads popping up all over the place it seems, with a new one becoming the latest craze almost every week. What we need, though, is a long-term solution, a lifestyle change that can get us back on track.

And that brings us back to not eating. What we're talking about here is not avoiding food altogether, but avoiding it for periods of time. It's called intermittent fasting, and while some people may call it another one of those weight-loss fads, it's more of a lifestyle change.

Intermittent fasting follows the practice of our forefathers, the earliest humans, who certainly didn't eat three meals a day and then have snacks in between while they sat at their computer or took a break at work. These humans, who were quite healthy from a physical standpoint, went long periods of time without eating as they either braved winter months of fewer abundance of plants to eat or searched for their next hunt.

Intermittent fasting is based on those principles, and as we'll soon see, it has wonderful, proven benefits for the human body, helping us to live longer and correcting some of the ills of unhealthy eating, such as low testosterone levels.

What is intermittent fasting?

Intermittent fasting is the practice of not eating for a set period of time each day. This practice may be in stark contrast to a lot of the weight-loss and healthy-eating programs out there that say you're supposed to eat small meals constantly throughout the day to promote metabolism. However, intermittent fasting has proven to have huge health benefits for humans.

73

When you are not consuming food, you are allowing your body to process the foods you do eat in a healthy way, over a time period that your body was built to withstand, from an evolutionary standpoint. Again, remember that our bodies are constructed the way they are today because of how our ancestors, the earliest humans, lived without food for long periods of time.

Fasting has also been used for centuries in spiritual and religious practices all over the world, in Christianity, Buddhism, Judaism and Islam.

Because it does not put restrictions on the types of foods you eat but rather when you eat them, intermittent fasting is considered an eating pattern more than it is a diet of healthy eating plan. And this eating pattern can actually be accomplished a few different ways.

One way of intermittent fasting is called the 5:2 method. Following this method means you will eat normally for five days a week, and then fast for the other two days of the week. Don't worry, though, you won't be fasting completely. On your two "fast days," whenever they may be, you should still eat, but keep your overall calorie intake between 500 and 600.

The next method is a slight variation on the 5:2, and it's called the eat-stop-eat method. Once or twice a week, you're supposed to fast completely for a 24-hour period, and then eat normally the rest of the week. If you decide to go this route and fast completely for two days each week, it's advisable that you don't make the fasting days back-to-back, otherwise you'll actually be fasting for 48 hours, which won't be good.

Then there is the 16/8 method, which integrates fasting into your daily routine. In this method, you are supposed to consume all of your calories for the day within a six- to eight-hour window, and then fast for the other 14 to 16 hours in a day. If you think about it, it's not that outlandish. Simply eat in the hours for which most people work – over a typical eight-hour workday. This is why the 16/8 method is one of the more popular methods of intermittent fasting.

While the types of food you eat aren't restricted in any of the intermittent fasting methods, you still shouldn't go out and stuff your face with a lot of bad foods. That would counteract all the good you're doing to your body by following an inter-mittent fasting program in the first place. You should try to eat as healthy as you can, or at least as close to as healthy as you can, in the periods in which you are supposed to eat per the method you choose.

A great way to make your intermittent fasting method work even better is to limit your carb intake. This is because doing so helps your body remain in a "fasting state," even though you are consuming foods.

The best part about intermittent fasting is that it won't prohibit you from drinking liquids – as long as it's water, coffee, tea and other zero-calorie beverages without sugar added – and it's OK to take supplements and exercise while following the eating pattern as well.

What are the benefits of intermittent fasting?

No matter which method of intermittent fasting you choose, you will be doing your body and your brain a lot of good. That's because all of these methods are designed to reduce your overall calorie intake, which will result in weight loss and an overall healthier body, and a longer-lasting life.

Studies have shown that an intermittent fasting practice can result in an increase in your body's metabolic rate by as much as 14 percent. Another study found that intermittent fasting can result in weight loss of 3-8 percent over only three to 24 weeks. That means a 200-pound person could lose up to 16 pounds in 24 weeks just by following this eating pattern. And that number could skyrocket even more if he or she makes sure to eat healthy foods in the time periods they are allowed to eat.

But intermittent fasting won't just result in the loss of body weight. It can also help you increase your lean body mass. Recent research has run in contrast to past research that said your body needed four to six meals per day to increase metabolism. This more recent research has proven that diets that are not restricted by calories but instead restrict the times during which you eat improve lean body mass, fat loss and overall weight loss.

But what are the benefits of intermittent fasting? Generally speaking, intermittent fasting can boost weight loss, increase your energy, promote cellular repair, reduce insulin resistance and protect against type 2 diabetes, lower bad cholesterol, promote longevity, improve memory and boost brain function.

When you fast, your body is going through a lot of changes. One of the things it does is adjust your hormone levels to make stored body fat more accessible. When it's more accessible, the fat ends up getting used in the proper ways it should, and it ends up getting burned off instead of unnecessarily stored for "future use." That process is the basis behind losing weight.

When you fast, your body is doing a lot. One of the main things that happens is that your levels of growth hormone go through the roof, increasing by almost five times. This has a significant impact on fat loss and also muscle gain.

When you fast, your insulin sensitivity improves, leading to lower levels of insulin in your body and again allowing that stored fat to be more easily accessible.

When you fast, you allow the cells in your body to repair themselves. This is an essential function of your body, but it's one that gets diminished if you're constantly eating.

When you fast, your genes start to function a little differently. These changes in gene expression have proven benefits such as longevity and protection against serious diseases.

Can intermittent fasting boost testosterone?

As we discussed already, intermittent fasting has been shown to have a significant effect on boosting levels of human growth hormone and the male growth hormone. This is the result of a dip in the body's blood sugar levels and an uptick in testosterone levels.

This is because testosterone is positively correlated with insulin sensitivity. Put more plainly, healthy insulin levels result in healthy testosterone levels.

As a result of this, if you're following an intermittent fasting plan because, in some fashion, you're looking to boost your testosterone levels, it is suggested that you ignore the suggestions of many and actually skip breakfast. This is because insulin levels are most sensitive in the morning, and your body also experiences a spike in cortisol levels after you wake up.

When you eat in the morning, what happens is that the food combines with these natural fats to rapidly decrease your blood glucose, resulting in what is referred to as false hunger, which then makes you eat more than you really need to. Skipping breakfast, then, helps you regulate your blood glucose levels, your insulin and your cortisol right from the get-go.

Intermittent fasting also increases the body's level of luteinizing hormone and overall testosterone levels. One study, in fact, found that intermittent fasting by non-obese men resulted in LH levels increasing by up to 67 percent and overall testosterone levels by up to 180 percent.

Remember, LH is what triggers the production of testosterone, so having a healthy and balanced LH level will naturally result in a higher level of testosterone. Intermittent fasting will cause your body to stimulate the production of hormones that are most associated with testosterone production. Let's not forget that testosterone itself is a hormone, so if your body is able to produce all its necessary hormones better, it will more easily be able to produce higher levels of testosterone and then utilize that testosterone in a more effective way.

Intermittent fasting also helps boost testosterone by the simple fact that your body will be burning fat and losing weight. One of the most natural ways to boost your testosterone level is to simply lose that excess body fat. When your body is losing weight, it is burning your excess body fat, using it for energy instead of storing it, and ridding itself of toxins. That's why intermittent fasting and testosterone levels are so related to each other.

In doctor-speak, testosterone levels are inversely correlated with insulin resistance and body fat levels. This means that as one goes up, the other goes down. So if your body fat levels are high, then your testosterone levels will go down. If your body fat levels go down, then, your testosterone levels will go up. It's as simple as that. And the best part is that both your free testosterone levels will increase through this loss of body fat, too, and not just the level of testosterone that's bound to other things, such as sex hormone-binding globulin.

Here's another interesting fact about testosterone and eating that we haven't touched on yet. Every time you eat something, your testosterone levels drop, and this happens no matter what you eat – whether it's super healthy or super unhealthy. This, then, would only naturally go to prove that eating meals more often throughout the day, even if those meals are small and healthy, would work in direct contrast to you if you're trying to boost your testosterone levels.

Rather, following a method of eating four to six meals a day would actually decrease your testosterone levels just by the nature of how your body works. That's another simple reason why intermittent fasting boosts testosterone levels. Eating in shorter windows of time each day limits the amount of time that your hormone levels are being negatively affected.

In another recent study, researchers analyzed the body before and after a 24-hour period of fasting. What they found was that after consuming no calories for 24 hours, participants' growth hormone levels had increased 2,000 percent. This just goes to show you the power of actually not eating.

What intermittent fasting does, at its core, is it not only helps increase testosterone indirectly by resulting in a loss of body fat, but intermittent fasting also increases testosterone directly by triggering both the production and the release of the all-important hormone.

What's the best way to do an intermittent fast?

Now that we have seen the tremendous benefits of intermittent fasting for longevity, testosterone levels and overall health, it's time to discuss what the best way to follow an intermittent fasting program, and who should do so.

As we talked about before, one of the most popular methods of intermittent fasting is the 16/8 method. This method says you consume all of your calories within an eight-hour window each day, and then fast for the remaining 16 hours of the day.

By design, the 16/8 method is probably the easiest intermittent fasting method for most people to follow. A suggestion is to start eating at noon and stop eating at 8 p.m. This means you will skip breakfast – giving you those significant benefits we talked about before – and begin eating around a typical lunchtime. This also gives you the added benefit of having a nice dinner at home with your family after work, and maybe even a small snack after.

That will leave your 16 fasting hours to be from 8 p.m. to noon the following day. If you think about it, that's not that hard to do. Possibly half of those hours will be taken up by sleeping anyway, and the more sleep you get, the better your body will be able to function the next day.

So, in reality, if go to sleep at 10 p.m. and wake up at 6 a.m., you'll only truly be fasting for eight waking hours – from 6 a.m. to noon and again from 8 p.m. to 10 p.m. That's not too bad at all. In addition, you are allowed to consume calorie-free liquids during your fasting periods. This includes water, plain tea, black coffee and other zero-calorie beverages. Make sure you don't add any sugar or milk to any of these beverages, and make sure to drink plenty of water throughout the day as well.

While the specific types of food you eat aren't technically restricted when you are following an intermittent fasting program, paying attention to what you consume during your eating hours and focusing on certain foods and drinks will help you have even better results.

The first suggestion is to eat lots of high-fiber foods when you are following an intermittent fast. That's because eating foods that are high in fiber, and also high in protein, will help to suppress your hunger. This will result in you not wanting to run to the pantry or the fridge when you are supposed to be fasting. Some of the best high-fiber foods are nuts, fruits and vegetables and beans. Some of the best high-protein foods are obviously meat, fish, tofu and actually nuts as well.

It's also important that when you are choosing your protein-rich foods that you opt for lean proteins whenever possible. That means turkey and chicken should be some of your top choices. When you choose to eat red meat, which is an OK option, try to go for the less fatty versions. There are plenty available and they are still delicious and satisfying.

Another thing to do when your following an intermittent fasting plan is to make sure you drink a lot of water. That's because our mind can often mistake being thirsty for being hungry. Doctors recommend that you should drink about half an ounce to an ounce of water for each pound you weigh. That means a 200-pound person should drink, on average, 150 ounces of water per day. That's more than a gallon of water each day. When you drink that much water, you'll actually be tricking your body into thinking it's full, helping to suppress your hunger.

As mentioned before, it's not only allowed but encouraged that you exercise when you are following an intermittent fasting plan. Exercise does your body good no matter what your eating habits, and intermittent fasting is no exception.

While doing an intermittent fast, it may be best for you to exercise in the mornings, if you can. That's because people get hungry about a half an hour or so after they exercise. If you aren't able to eat soon after you exercise, then it might be harder for you to stick to the eating schedule. Just think, if you are following the 16/8 plan and exercise at 9 p.m., you might get hungry around 10 p.m. but not be able to eat for 14 more hours.

No matter which method you choose, and which food, drink and exercise regiments you decide to integrate into that method, intermittent fasting is a great, proven and effective way of increasing your longevity and boosting your testosterone levels, all while resulting in an overall healthier you.